Atkins Diet

Cookbook

Breakfast Recipes

54 Easy and Delicious Recipes to Help You Lose Weight and Improve Your Health

Maggie Vega

Table of Contents

3

Introduction

What is the Atkins Diet?

It is basically a low-carbs diet termed as Atkins Diet after the name of the physician Dr. Robert C. Atkins who promoted it in the year 1972. He also wrote a book in the same year to guide people with the diet.

The Atkins diet allows minimum intake of the carbohydrates so that body's metabolism boosts which helps in the burning of body's fat to produce energy and body undergo a process of ketosis. Ketosis process starts with the lower insulin levels in the body causing the consumption and burning of the fats to generate ketone bodies. On contrary, consumption of higher carbohydrates increases blood sugar levels thus accumulation of the fats occurs.

Atkins diet promotes simple eating habits which reduces the appetite. Atkins diet foods are rich in fats and proteins thus longer duration of digestion is required which lowers the raise of hunger.

Formerly, the Atkins diet was considered unhealthy because of the high saturated fat intake but recent research has proved it harmless. In fact the high consumption of high fat diet like Atkins diet has shown tremendous health improvements like lowering the blood sugar levels, cholesterol levels, triglycerides and makes you tidy up to look smarter and fresh. The main reason that is most appealing to use this diet is that it is helpful in lowering done your appetite which vanishes with a little intake of calories.

The Atkins Diet Plan

The Atkins diet is usually split up into 4 different phases with each phase with different food items:

Induction phase (phase 1): This phase of the diet is quite tough as one has to intake less than 20 grams of carbs each day for 2 weeks. High proteins and fats are encouraged to eat with leaf green vegetables that contain low carbohydrates. These healthy weeks will start your weight loss.

Balancing Phase (phase 2): In this phase, try to create a equilibrium in your diet by slowly adding low-carb vegetables, more nuts, and a little amount of fruit back in your food.

1. Fine-Tuning Phase (phase 3): Seeing yourself near the required goal or optimum weight you want then slowly add more carbohydrates in the diet plan to slow down the further weight loss now.

2. Maintenance Phase (phase 4): Each as much carbs as much you can but keep it in mind that the body shouldn't regain the weight. Excess of everything is bad.

A number of people skip the induction phase and intake lots of fruits and vegetables at the beginning that can be effective too. Other do prefer induction phase to activate ketosis process which is low-carb keto diet.

Foods for Atkins Diet:

People usually get confused what should be eating during the diet and what should not... an outlines of food is listed below:

Prohibited food:

Try to avoid the mentioned food items while you are on the Atkins diet plan:

Grains: Spelt, rye, Wheat, barley, rice.

Sugar: Fruit juices, cakes, Soft drinks, candy, ice cream, etc

Vegetable Oils: Soybean oil, cottonseed oil, corn oil, canola oil and many others.

Low-Fat Foods: foods those are rich in sugar content.

Trans Fats: The tin pack things with mentioning of hydrogenated ingredients on the list.

High-Carb Fruits: Apples, oranges, pears, bananas, grapes (while in induction

phase).

Starches: Sweet potatoes, Potatoes (for induction phase only).

High-Carb Vegetables: Turnips, Carrots, etc (for induction only).

Legumes: Lentils, chickpeas, beans.

Beneficial Food items:

Healthy food items like the following should be in your menu for the Atkins diet Seafood and Fatty Fish: Trout, Salmon, sardines, etc.

Meats: Lamb, chicken, Beef, pork, bacon and others.

Eggs: Eggs are rich in Omega-3.

Healthy Fats: Coconut oil, avocado oil and extra virgin olive oil.

Full-Fat Dairy: Butter, full-fat yoghurt, cheese, cream.

Low-Carb Vegetables: Spinach, broccoli, Kale, asparagus and others alike.

Nuts and Seeds: Macadamia nuts, sunflower seeds, almonds, walnuts, etc.

Recipes

1. SPINACH CHICKEN PARMESAN

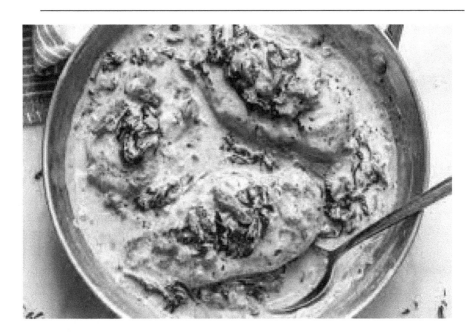

Ingredients:

- 1/3 cup grated Parmesan cheese
- 1/4 teaspoon Italian seasoning
- 6 skinless, boneless chicken breasts
- 1 tablespoon butter
- 1 tablespoon all-purpose flour
- 1/2 cup skim milk
- 1/2 (10 ounce) package frozen chopped spinach, thawed and drained

- 1 tablespoon chopped pimento peppers

Directions:

1. Preheat oven to 350 degrees F (175 degrees C).
2. In a small bowl combine cheese and seasoning. After that, roll chicken pieces in cheese mixture to coat lightly. Set remaining cheese mixture aside.
3. Then, arrange coated chicken pieces in an 8x8x2 inch baking dish.
4. In a small saucepan, saute green onion in butter/margarine until tender.
5. Next, stir in flour, then add milk all at once. Simmer, stirring, until bubbly.
6. Stir in drained spinach and pimiento and combine together.
7. Spoon spinach mixture over chicken and sprinkle with remaining cheese mixture.
8. After that, bake uncovered for 30 to 35 minutes or until tender and chicken juices run clear. Delicious!

2. LAZY TOMATO SALSA

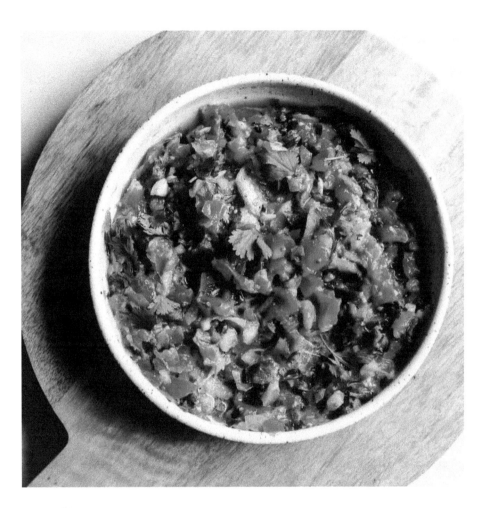

Ingredients:

- 3 tomatoes, chopped
- 1/2 cup finely diced onion
- 5 serrano chiles, finely chopped
- 1/2 cup chopped fresh cilantro

- 1 teaspoon salt

Directions:

1. In a mixing bowl, stir together tomatoes, onion, chili peppers, salt, and lime juice.
2. Then, chill for one hour in the refrigerator before serving.

3. HEARTY PAN-FRIED ASPARAGUS

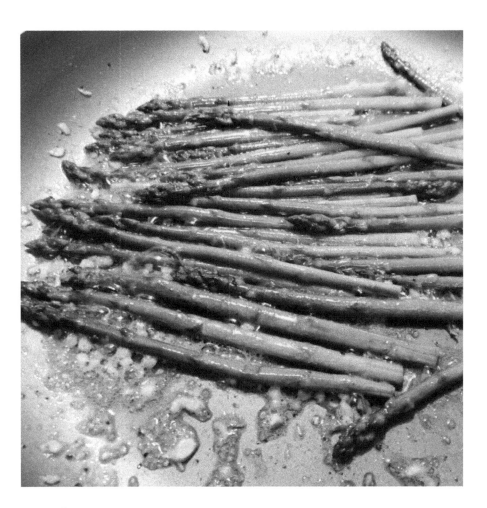

Ingredients:

- 1/4 cup butter
- 2 tablespoons olive oil
- 3 cloves garlic, minced
- 1 pound fresh asparagus spears, trimmed

- pepper to taste

Directions:

1. Melt butter in a skillet over medium-high heat.
2. Afterwards, stir in the olive oil, salt, and pepper.
3. Cook garlic in butter for a minute, but do not brown.
4. After that, add asparagus, and cook for 10 minutes, turning asparagus to ensure even cooking.

4. EGG AND CHEESE BOATS

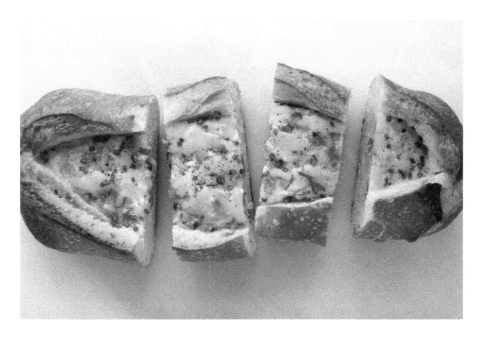

Ingredients:

- 2 oval sandwich rolls
- 4 eggs
- 3 tablespoons whole milk
- 1 (4 ounce) can chopped green chile peppers
- 1 cup shredded sharp Cheddar cheese
- 1/2 cup shredded pepper Jack cheese
- 1/2 teaspoon smoked paprika
- pepper to taste

Directions:

1. Preheat oven to 350 degrees F (175 degrees C). Next, line a rimmed baking sheet with parchment paper. Make a V-shaped cut in each roll, leaving the ends intact.
2. After that, lift out V-shaped wedge. Hollow out rolls gently to make shallow bread bowls, being careful not to cut through the bottom or sides.
3. Then, place bread bowls on the prepared baking sheet. Whisk eggs in a bowl. Add milk; whisk until well blended.
4. Stir in green chile peppers, Cheddar cheese, pepper Jack cheese, salt.
5. Next, pour mixture slowly into the prepared rolls, spreading evenly with a spoon.
6. After that, bake in the preheated oven until egg mixture is completely set and cheese is lightly browned, about 30 minutes.
7. Cool for 3 minutes before serving.

5. FAST CHICKEN STUFFED BAKED AVOCADOS

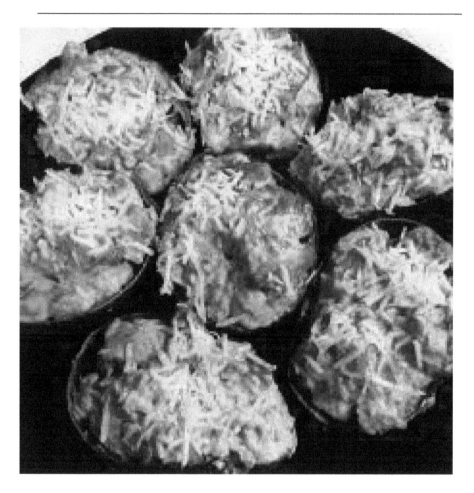

Ingredients:

- 4 avocados, halved and pitted
- 2 cooked chicken breasts, shredded
- 4 ounces cream cheese, softened
- 1/4 cup chopped tomatoes

- 1 pinch cayenne pepper
- 1/2 cup shredded Parmesan cheese, or more to taste
- salt to taste

Directions:

1. Preheat oven to 400 degrees F (200 degrees C).
2. Afterwards, scoop out some of the flesh in the center of each avocado; place into mixing bowl.
3. Now, add chicken, cream cheese, tomatoes, salt, cayenne pepper; mix nicely to combine.
4. Scoop spoonfuls of chicken mixture into the wells of each avocado; top each with generous amount of Parmesan cheese.
5. After that, place avocado halves, face-up, in muffin cups to stabilize.
6. Bake avocados in preheated oven until cheese is melted, 8 to 10 minutes.

6. THE BEST DEVILED EGGS

Ingredients:

- 6 eggs
- 1/4 cup mayonnaise
- 2 tablespoons finely chopped onion
- 3 tablespoons sweet pickle relish
- 1 tablespoon prepared horseradish
- 1 tablespoon prepared mustard
- paprika, for garnish
- pepper to taste

Directions:

1. Place eggs in a medium saucepan and cover with cold water.
2. Then, bring water to a boil and immediately remove from heat. After that, cover and let eggs stand in hot water for 10 to 12 minutes.
3. Remove from hot water, cool, peel and cut lengthwise.
4. Afterwards, remove yolks from eggs.
5. In a medium bowl, mash the yolks and mix together with mayonnaise, onion, horseradish and mustard.

6. With a fork or pastry bag, fill the egg halves with the yolk mixture.
7. Garnish with paprika, salt and pepper.
8. Chill until serving.

7. FAST DEVILED EGGS

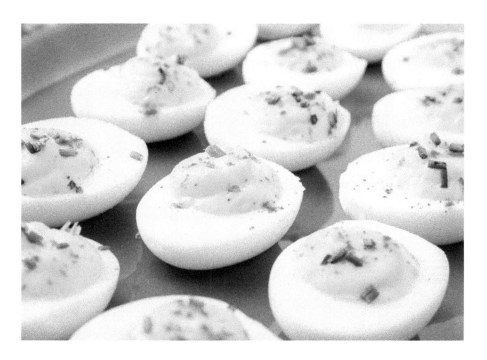

Ingredients:

- 6 eggs
- 1/2 teaspoon paprika
- 2 tablespoons mayonnaise
- 1/2 teaspoon mustard powder

Directions:

1. Place eggs in a pot of salted water.

2. Next, bring the water to a boil, and let eggs cook in boiling water until they are hard boiled, approximately 10 to 15 minutes.
3. Afterwards, drain eggs, and let cool.
4. Cut eggs in half, lengthwise.
5. Remove the egg yolks and mash them together in a small mixing bowl.
6. Combine in the paprika, mayonnaise, and dry mustard.
7. Spoon mixture into the egg whites; cool and serve.

8. MINI HAM AND CHEESE ROLLS

Ingredients:

- 2 tablespoons dried minced onion
- 1 tablespoon prepared mustard
- 2 tablespoons poppy seeds
- 1/2 cup margarine, melted
- 24 dinner rolls
- salt to taste
- 1/2 pound chopped ham
- 1/2 pound thinly sliced Swiss cheese

Instructions:

1. Preheat oven to 325 degrees F (165 degrees C).
2. In a mixing bowl, mix onion flakes, mustard, poppy seeds and margarine.
3. After that, split each dinner roll.
4. Make a sandwich of the ham and cheese and the dinner rolls.
5. Afterwards, arrange the sandwiches on a baking sheet.
6. Drizzle the poppy seed mixture over the sandwiches. Bake for 20 minutes, or until cheese has melted.
7. Serve these sandwiches warm.

9. CALIFORNIA CHICKEN

Ingredients:

- 4 skinless, boneless chicken breasts
- 1 teaspoon olive oil
- 1/2 teaspoon onion powder
- 1 pinch ground black pepper
- 2 avocados
- 2 ripe tomatoes, sliced
- 1 package Monterey Jack cheese
- salt

Instructions:

1. Preheat oven to 350 degrees F (175 degrees C).
2. Now, warm oil in skillet and add chicken and onion.
3. Cook 15 minutes or until chicken is browned and just about done.
4. Now, add salt and pepper to taste.
5. Place chicken on cookie sheet and top each breast with 1 to 2 slices of tomato and 2 to 3 slices of cheese.
6. Afterwards, place in oven for 10 to 15 minutes, until cheese melts.
7. Remove from oven, add 2 to 3 slices of avocado on top of each breast, and serve immediately.

10.   BABY SPINACH OMELET

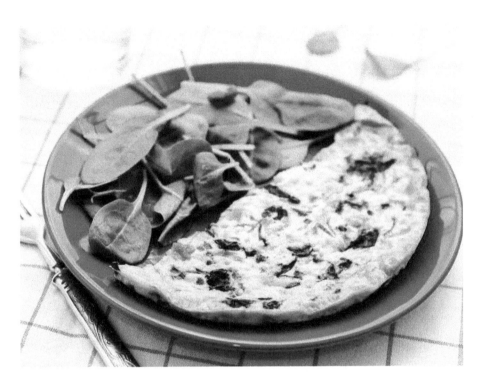

Ingredients:

- 2 eggs
- 1 cup torn baby spinach leaves
- 1 1/2 tablespoons grated Parmesan cheese
- 1/4 teaspoon onion powder
- 1/8 teaspoon ground nutmeg
- pepper to taste

Directions:

1. In a bowl, beat the eggs, and stir in the baby spinach and Parmesan cheese.

2. Then, season with onion powder, nutmeg, salt.

3. In a small skillet coated with cooking spray over medium heat, cook the egg mixture about 3 minutes, until partially set.

4. Next, flip with a spatula, and continue cooking 2 to 3 minutes.

5. Reduce heat to low, and continue cooking 2 to 3 minutes, or to desired doneness.

11.   FAST AVOCADO CORN SALSA

Ingredients:

- 1 (16 ounce) package frozen corn kernels
- 2 (2.25 ounce) cans sliced ripe olives
- 1 red bell pepper
- 1 small onion
- 5 cloves garlic
- 1/3 cup olive oil
- 1/4 cup lemon juice
- 1 teaspoon dried oregano
- 1/2 teaspoon salt
- 1/2 teaspoon ground black pepper
- 4 avocados

Directions:

1. In a large bowl, combine corn, olives, red bell pepper and onion.
2. Next, in a small bowl, combine garlic, olive oil, lemon juice, oregano, salt and pepper.
3. Then, pour into the corn mixture and toss to coat.
4. Cover and chill in the refrigerator 8 hours, or overnight.
5. Stir avocados into the mixture before serving.

12. COCONUT DIRTY CHAI LATTE

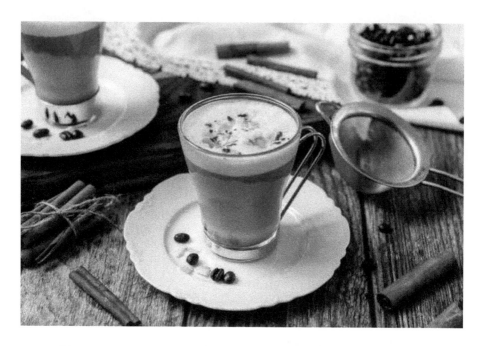

Ingredients:

- 1 cup brewed chai tea
- 1 cup warm coconut milk
- 1 teaspoon instant espresso powder
- 1/2 teaspoon ground cinnamon
- 1 teaspoon honey
- pepper to taste

Directions:

1. Mix chai tea, coconut milk, espresso powder, and cinnamon in a blender; blend until smooth.

2. Pour into 2 mugs; drizzle with honey and sprinkle with shredded coconut.

13. CREAMY CAULIFLOWER TORTILLAS

Ingredients:

- 1 head cauliflower, finely grated
- 2 eggs
- pepper to taste

Directions:

1. Preheat oven to 400 degrees F (200 degrees C). Line a baking sheet with parchment paper.
2. Place cauliflower in a microwave-safe bowl.
3. Microwave at maximum power until tender, about 4 minutes. Next, place on a kitchen towel and squeeze out all liquid; transfer to a bowl.
4. Whisk eggs, salt, and black pepper in a bowl. Add to the cauliflower in batches; stir well.
5. Shape cauliflower mixture into 3-inch tortillas on the prepared baking sheet. Bake in the preheated oven until set, about 20 minutes.
6. Let cool slightly.
7. Heat a skillet over medium heat. Cook tortillas until golden brown, about 1 minute.
8. Flip and cook for 1 minute more.

14. PEANUT BUTTER COOKIES

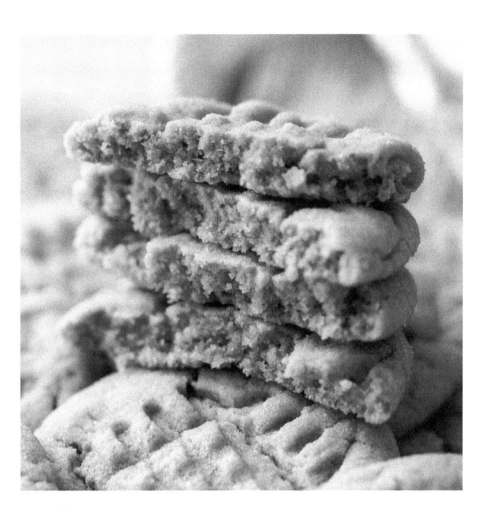

Ingredients:

- 1 cup peanut butter
- 1/2 cup low-calorie natural sweetener (such as Swerve(R))
- 1 egg
- 1 teaspoon sugar-free vanilla extract

Directions:

1. Preheat oven to 350 degrees F (175 degrees C). Line a baking sheet with parchment paper.
2. Combine peanut butter, sweetener, egg, and vanilla extract in a bowl; blend well until a dough is formed. Roll dough into 1-inch balls.
3. Place on the prepared baking sheet and press down twice with a fork in a criss-cross pattern.
4. Afterwards, bake in the preheated oven until edges are golden, 12 to 15 minutes.
5. Cool on the baking sheet for 1 minute before removing to a wire rack to cool completely.

15.   CHEESE CRISPS

Ingredients:

- 1 cup shredded Cheddar cheese

Directions:

1. Preheat oven to 400 degrees F (200 degrees C).
2. Line 2 baking sheets with parchment paper.
3. Arrange Cheddar cheese in 24 small heaps on the prepared baking sheets.
4. After that, bake in the preheated oven until golden brown, about 7 minutes.
5. Cool for 5 to 10 minutes before removing from baking sheets.

16.   FLUFFY PANCAKES

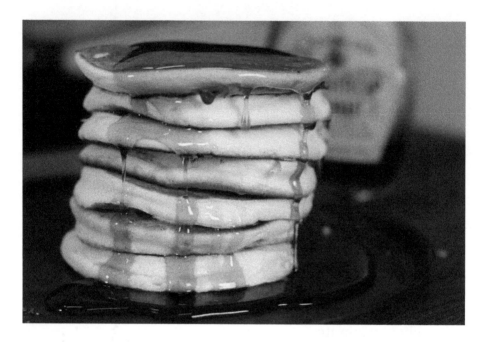

Ingredients:

- 1 cup almond flour
- 1/4 cup coconut flour
- 2 tablespoons low-calorie natural sweetener
- 1 teaspoon baking powder
- 6 eggs, at room temperature
- 1/4 cup heavy whipping cream
- 2 tablespoons butter, melted
- 1 teaspoon vanilla extract
- salt to taste

Directions:

1. Mix almond flour, coconut flour, sweetener, salt, baking powder, and cinnamon together in a bowl.
2. Whisk in eggs, heavy cream, butter, and vanilla extract slowly until batter is just blended.
3. Heat a lightly oiled griddle over medium-high heat.
4. Then, drop batter by large spoonful onto the griddle and cook until bubbles form and the edges are dry, 3 to 4 minutes.
5. Flip and cook until browned on the other side, 2 to 3 minutes.
6. Repeat with remaining batter.

17. CHOCOLATE-PEANUT BUTTER CUPS

Ingredients:

- 1 cup coconut oil
- 1/2 cup natural peanut butter
- 2 tablespoons heavy cream
- 1 tablespoon cocoa powder
- 1 teaspoon liquid stevia
- 1/4 teaspoon vanilla extract
- 1 ounce chopped roasted salted peanuts

Directions:

1. Melt coconut oil in a saucepan over low heat, 3 to 5 minutes.
2. Stir in peanut butter until smooth. Afterwards, whisk in heavy cream, cocoa powder, liquid stevia, vanilla extract, and salt.
3. Pour chocolate-peanut butter mixture into 12 silicone muffin molds.
4. Sprinkle peanuts evenly on top. Place molds on a baking sheet.
5. Freeze chocolate-peanut butter mixture until firm, at least 1 hour.

6. Unmold chocolate-peanut cups and transfer to a resealable plastic bag or airtight container.

18. OMELET WITH AVOCADO

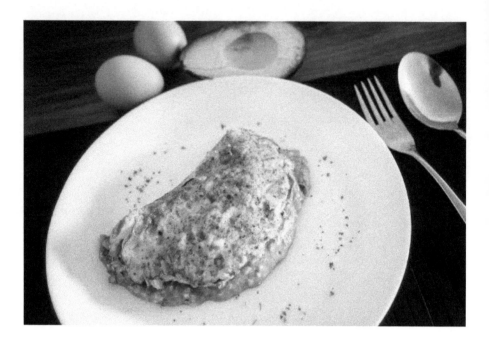

- Ingredients
- 2 eggs (large)
- 1 tablespoon coconut oil or butter
- 2 tablespoons of water
- ½ avocado
- 1 serving pepper jack or cheddar cheese
- 1 tablespoon salsa (for topping)

Directions:

1. Beating the Eggs Start off by cracking two eggs into a bowl and adding 2 tablespoons of water.
2. Add salt and pepper to taste and whisk the eggs with a fork or hand whisk until the whites and yolks are thoroughly blended together.
3. Making the Omelet
4. Get out a nonstick skillet and pour in a tablespoon of butter or coconut oil, depending on your preference.
5. Heat the skillet on medium-high and note that the oil or butter will get hot very quickly.
6. Once the butter has melted, pour in the egg mixture.
7. You'll see that the mixture should start to set immediately.
8. Grab your spatula and gently pull all of the sides of the mixture toward the center.
9. When the edges are set but the inside is still soft, you're ready to add your filling ingredients.
10. For this recipe, just add cheese.

19.   SCRAMBLED EGGS WITH SALMON

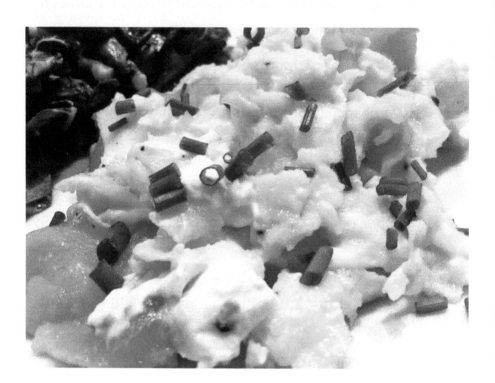

Ingredients

- 4 eggs
- 1 tablespoon milk or heavy cream
- Salt and pepper to taste
- 1 tablespoon butter
- ¼ pound smoked salmon, sliced OR ½ pound sautéed salmon fillet cut into cubes
- Dill or chive to taste (optional)

Directions:

1. Starting the Eggs
2. In a small bowl, whisk together the eggs, milk or heavy cream, salt and pepper.
3. Meanwhile, melt the butter in a nonstick skillet on medium high heat.
4. When the butter is melted, add in the egg mixture and use a wooden spoon or spatula to push around the eggs.
5. Adding the Salmon
6. While the cooking eggs still have a wet texture, add in the salmon.
7. You can use canned, smoked or cooked salmon chunks according to your preference.
8. Stir the salmon into the eggs and continue scrambling them until they're cooked to your liking.

20.   STEAK AND EGGS

Ingredients

- 8 ounces of flank steak (avoid cuts of steaks with excess amounts of fat or trim if needed)
- 1 tablespoon olive oil or butter
- 2-4 eggs
- 1 ounce of shredded cheese (pepper-jack works well)
- 1 tablespoon salsa (for topping)

Directions:

1. Cooking the steak In a large nonstick skillet, heat butter until foaming and melted on high heat.
2. Season the steak with salt and pepper to your liking and place in the skillet.
3. Instead of putting butter in the pan, you can also coat the steak with cooking spray (just make sure to choose butter-based cooking sprays without additives).
4. Reduce the heat and cook the steak for about 15 minutes, turning as needed to brown both sides.
5. Alternatively, you can sear the steak on high heat and then transfer it to an oven preheated to 350 degrees Fahrenheit.

Cook it in the oven for about 5 minutes until desired doneness (use a meat thermometer).

6. Once the steak is cooked, put it
7. onto a cutting board to rest and wipe out the excess juices from the skillet.
8. Cooking the Eggs
9. Using the same skillet, cook the eggs in any way you'd like.
10. To cook them sunny side up, simply crack the eggs into a skillet heated to high heat for about 3 minutes.
11. Scrambled also pairs well with the steak.

21. BELGIAN WAFFLES

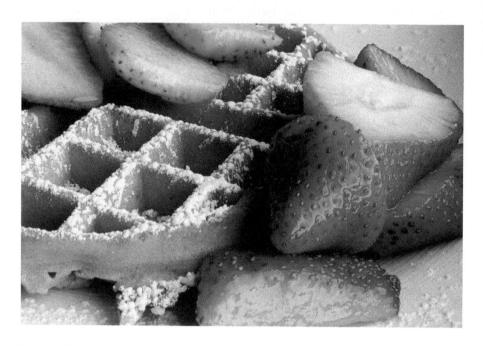

Ingredients:

- 1 cup bake mix
- 1 Tbsp baking powder
- 3 packets sugar substitute
- 1 tsp salt
- ¼ cup heavy cream
- 3 eggs
- 1 tsp vanilla
- ½ cup ice water

Instructions:

1. Heat a waffle iron. Whisk together the bake mix, baking powder, sugar substitute and salt.

2. Add cream, eggs, vanilla extract and ice water.

3. Pour in a little more water if necessary, 1 tablespoon at a time, until batter spreads easily.

4. Place approximately 3 tablespoons batter in center of waffle iron.

5. Cook according to manufacturer's directions until crisp and dark golden brown.

6. Repeat with remaining batter.

22.   FLAXSEED PANCAKE

Ingredients:

- 1 pinch cinnamon
- 1 tsp vanilla
- 2 tsp baking powder
- 6 Tbsp ground flax seed
- 1 cup egg beaters

Instructions:

1. Pour egg beaters into a bowl.

2. Add the remaining ingredients into the bowl. Mix well.

3. Set aside for 1 minute then mix again.

4. Put a skillet over medium heat and spray with oil.

5. Divide pancake mixture into four batches. Cook each batch as you would a regular pancake.

23. WHOLE-WHEAT CURRANT SCONES

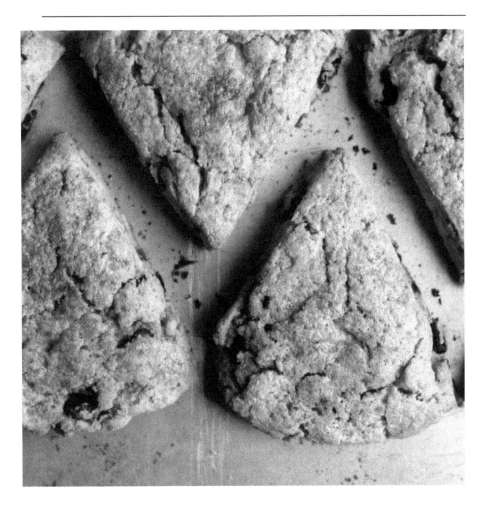

Ingredients:

- ¼ cup currants
- 1 cup whole-wheat flour
- 1 cup Atkins Cuisine All Purpose Baking Mix
- 2 Tbsp granular sugar substitute

- 4 tsp baking powder
- 2 tsp ground ginger
- ⅛ tsp ground nutmeg
- ⅛ tsp salt
- 5 Tbsp cold unsalted butter, cut into pieces
- 2 large eggs, lightly beaten
- ¾ cup heavy cream

Instructions:

1.Heat oven to 400°F. Soak currants for 15 minutes in a cup of warm water.

2.Pulse flour, baking mix, sugar substitute, baking powder, ginger, nutmeg, and salt in a food processor. Add butter; pulse until well combined. Add eggs and heavy cream; pulse for 2 minutes. Drain currants and add; pulse until just combined.

3.Drop ¼-cup mounds on an ungreased baking sheet; press gently to flatten slightly. Bake until lightly golden, about 10 minutes.

4.Serve warm or at room temperature.

24. PEANUT-STRAWBERRY BREAKFAST BARS

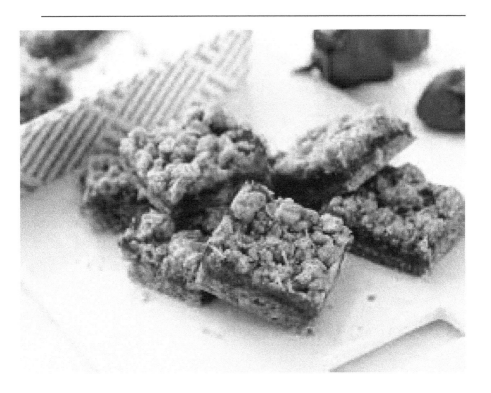

Ingredients:

- Olive oil cooking spray
- 1¼ cups old-fashioned rolled oats
- 1¼ cups granular sugar substitute
- ½ cup all purpose baking mix
- ¼ cup whole-wheat flour
- ¼ tsp salt
- ½ cup (1 stick) unsalted butter, melted

- 3 large eggs, lightly beaten
- ¾ cup unsweetened natural peanut butter
- ½ cup no-sugar-added strawberry jam

Instructions:

1. Heat oven to 350°F. Mist a 7-by-11-inch baking dish with cooking spray.
2. Mix oats, sugar substitute, baking mix, flour, and salt in a medium bowl; stir in butter and eggs until well combined.
3. Spread out half the dough in the baking dish.
4. Spread peanut butter evenly over dough; spread preserves evenly over peanut butter.
5. Crumble remaining dough over preserves.
6. Bake for about 25 minutes.
7. Cool completely before cutting into 12 pieces.

25. CRUNCHY TROPICAL BERRY AND ALMOND BREAKFAST PARFAIT

Ingredients:

- ½ cup heavy cream
- 1½ tsp granular sugar substitute, divided
- ¼ tsp coconut extract or pure vanilla extract
- ½ cup plain unsweetened whole-milk Greek yogurt
- 1 cup raspberries
- 1 cup blueberries or sliced strawberries
- 8 Tbsp Sweet and Salty Almonds
- ½ cup unsweetened shredded coconut, toasted

Instructions:

1. Combine cream, ½ tsp sugar substitute, and coconut extract or vanilla extract in a medium bowl; whip with an electric mixer for 3 minutes.
2. Add in the yogurt.
3. Mix raspberries and remaining sugar substitute in a blender until smooth.

4. In 4 parfait glasses, alternate layers of whipped cream, raspberry purée, blueberries, nuts, and shredded coconut, making two layers of each.

5. Serve right away.

26. CAULIFLOWER RICE SCRAMBLES

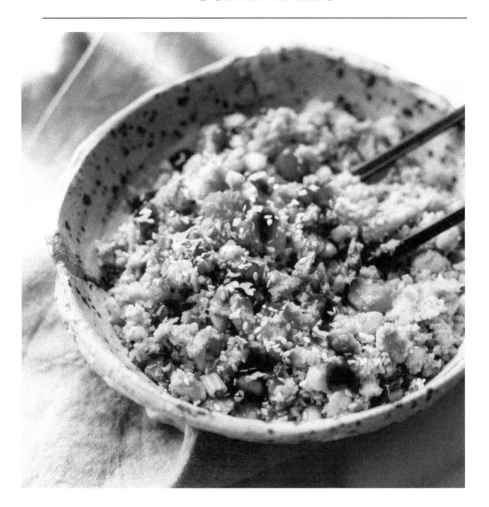

Ingredients:

- 1 head cauliflower, cut into florets (about 5 cups)
- 8 slices bacon
- 2 jalapeños, seeded and diced
- 8 large eggs

- 1 cup shredded cheddar cheese
- Hot sauce, to taste

Instructions:

1. Chop the cauliflower florets roughly in a food processor.
2. Warm the bacon in a large skillet over medium heat, and cook 4 to 5 minutes, stirring occasionally.
3. Transfer to a plate.
4. Do not discard the bacon grease.
5. Add the cauliflower and jalapeños to the bacon grease in the skillet, and cook 5 to 6 minutes, stirring often, until the cauliflower is soft.
6. Place the eggs and cheddar in a large bowl, and gently whisk. Add the eggs to the skillet and cook 3 to 4 minutes, stirring occasionally, until firm. Serve immediately with the bacon and hot sauce, if desired.

27.   BROILER HUEVOS RANCHEROS

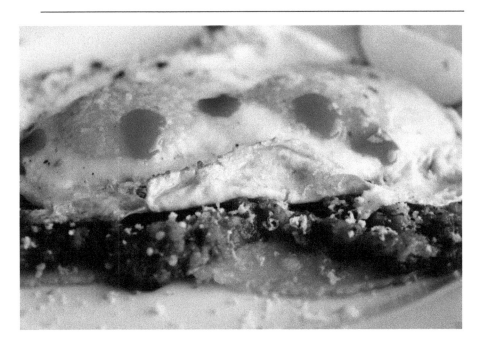

Ingredients:

- Olive oil spray
- 2 chorizo sausage links, (about 6 ounces) thinly sliced
- 1 bunch asparagus, trimmed and chopped
- 2 cups broccoli florets
- 2 cups cauliflower florets
- 8 large eggs
- ½ cup commercial tomato salsa
- 1 ripe Hass avocado, cut into wedges
- ¼ cup sour cream

Instructions:

1. Set the oven to broil and coat a large skillet with olive oil spray.

2. Place over medium heat and add the chorizo, browning for 3 to 4 minutes, stirring well, until it renders its fat.

3. Add the asparagus, broccoli, and cauliflower, and cook 3 to 4 minutes, until the vegetables start to soften.

4. Crack the eggs on top.

5. Cook under the broiler on the middle oven rack for 3 to 4 minutes.

6. Serve immediately with the salsa, avocado, and sour cream.

28. CHEESE PANCAKE

Ingredients:

- 1 Tbsp ground flax seed
- ½ tsp ground cinnamon
- 1 packet Stevia
- 4 oz cream cheese
- 2 eggs

Instructions:

1. Whisk the egg whites in a bowl.
2. In a separate bowl, beat the cream cheese with an electric mixer until smooth.
3. Combine the egg yolk with the cream cheese.
4. Add the flax seed, salt, stevia and cinnamon.
5. Continue to beat the mixture.
6. Fold in the beaten egg whites.
7. Put a pan over medium heat and add a small amount of butter.
8. Scoop ¼ cup from the mixture.
9. Cook the pancake for 3 minutes or until golden brown.
10. Then, serve.

29. CRANBERRY-ORANGE LOAF

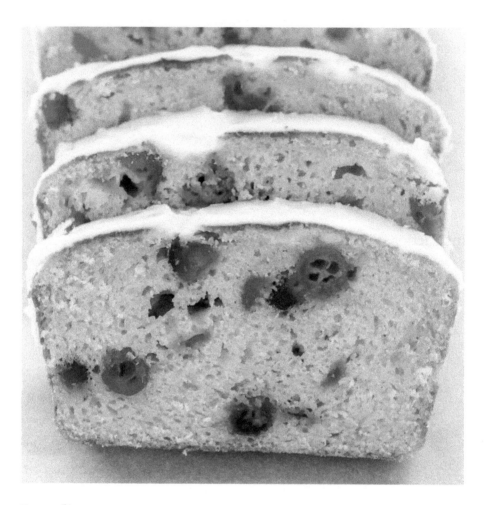

Ingredients:

- 1 cup fresh or frozen cranberries, thawed
- 1¼ cups Atkins Bake Mix
- ½ cup walnuts, toasted and ground
- 16 packets sugar substitute

- 1 tsp baking soda
- ½ tsp salt
- 1 stick (8 Tbsp) butter, softened
- 2 Tbsp sour cream
- 2 eggs
- 1 Tbsp grated fresh orange zest
- 1 tsp vanilla extract
- 2 egg whites

Instructions:

1. Heat oven to 350°F Grease a 9-inch-by-5-inch loaf pan; set aside.
2. Coarsely chop cranberries; set aside. In a medium bowl, mix walnuts, sugar substitute, bake mix, baking soda and salt until combined.
3. In another bowl, beat butter 3 minutes with an electric mixer on medium, until fluffy.
4. Beat in sour cream, eggs, orange zest and vanilla extract. Fold in cranberries.
5. Combine together the bake mix mixture and butter mixture. In another bowl,
6. beat egg whites for about 2 minutes. In three portions, fold egg whites into batter.
7. Spoon batter into prepared pan. Bake 50 to 55 minutes.
8. Cool on wire rack.
9. Cut loaf into thin slices.

30. PANCAKES WITH RICOTTA-APRICOT FILLING

Ingredients:

- 3 eggs
- 3 Tbsp Atkins Bake Mix
- ¼ tsp salt
- ⅓ cup heavy cream;
- ¾ cup ricotta cheese
- ¼ cup sugar-free apricot jam
- 1 packet sugar substitute
- 1½ Tbsp butter

Instructions:

1. In a bowl, whisk eggs, bake mix and salt until smooth.
2. Gradually whisk in cream.
3. Set aside for 5 minutes.
4. Press ricotta through a fine sieve into a bowl.
5. Mix in jam and sugar substitute.
6. Melt butter in a nonstick skillet over medium heat.
7. Pour in 2 tablespoons batter and tilt skillet to coat bottom.
8. Cook until golden on bottom; turn over.
9. Cook 1 minute more.
10. Transfer to a plate.

11. Repeat with remaining batter. Spread pancakes with ricotta mixture, roll up and serve

31. ATKINS YORKSHIRE PUDDING

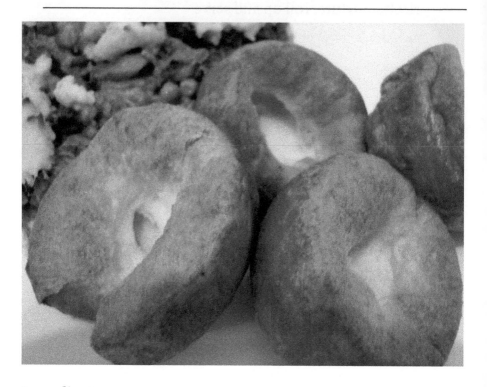

Ingredients:

- ½ cup Atkins Bake Mix
- ¼ cup wheat gluten
- 3 eggs
- 1 cup whole milk
- 1 tsp salt
- ⅓ cup beef drippings or vegetable oil

Instructions:

1. Heat oven to 450°F. Whisk together bake mix, gluten, eggs, milk and salt.
2. Pour drippings or oil into a muffin tin (½ tbsp each); place on centre rack in oven for 10 minutes, until smoky hot.
3. Add batter; bake 15 minutes.
4. Lower temperature to 350°F; cook 20 minutes more, until lightly browned.
5. Serve warm.

32.   BIRDIES IN A BASKET

Ingredients:

- 1 Tbsp olive oil
- ½ bunch asparagus, trimmed and sliced
- ½ tsp seasoning salt
- 2 large green bell peppers, halved crosswise, seeded
- 4 large eggs
- 2 cups shredded cheddar cheese

Instructions:

1. Heat a skillet, and add the olive oil.
2. Add the asparagus and seasoning salt; cook 3 to 4 minutes, until the asparagus softens.
3. Transfer to a plate.
4. Preheat the oven to 350°F. Place the peppers in the skillet, stem side down, and sear for 1 minute over medium heat.
5. Flip and crack an egg into each pepper half.
6. Top with the asparagus and sprinkle with the cheddar.
7. Bake for 30 minutes, the whites of the eggs are cooked through.
8. Serve immediately.

33.   GREEN EGGS AND HAM

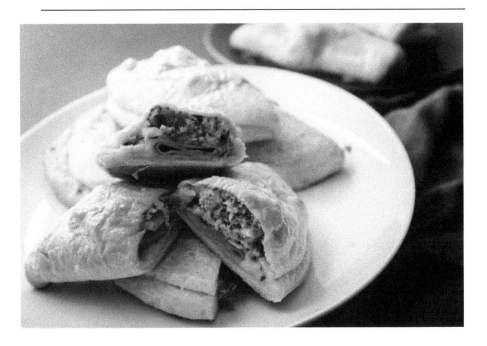

Ingredients:

- 2 eggs
- 1/4 - 1/2 avacado
- salt and pepper slices of ham (or bacon)

Directions:

1. Hard boil the eggs and mash or chop them up while still warm.
2. Mix with the avocado to make a green egg salad.
3. Add salt and pepper to taste.
4. Lightly fry the slices of ham and serve with the egg salad.

5. I like to use the egg salad chilled and roll it up in slices of cold ham like a crepe.

34. SWISS CANADIAN BACON AND EGGS

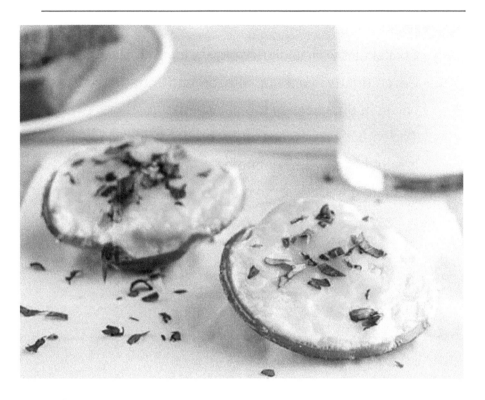

Ingredients:

- 8 large eggs
- 1/4 cup milk
- 1/2 tea. Salt
- 1/4 tea. Pepper
- 1/3 cups finely chopped green onion, divided
- 4 oz swiss cheese

Directions:

1. Preheat broiler in medium mixing bowl whisk together eggs, milk, salt and pepper until well blended.

2. Stir in all but 2 tbl onions place 12" skillet over med-low heat until hot.

3. Coat skillet with cooking spray, add egg mixture.

4. Cover tightly; cook 14 min or until almost set arrange bacon in pinwheel on top of egg mixture.

5. Top with cheese; place under broiler 2 min or until cheese is bubbly; top with remaining 2tbls onion.

6. Cut into 4 wedges serve immediately

35. PANCAKES OR WAFFLES

Ingredients:

- 1/2 cup Atkins Bake Mix;
- 1/4 cup FlaxSeed Meal (I used Bob's Red Mill w 0 net carbs);
- 1/4 cp Splenda (their website says the body does not recognize it as carbs);
- 1 egg- beaten;
- 3/4 cup water;
- 1/4 cup canola oil;1/2 tsp soda;
- 1 tsp baking powder;
- 1/4 cup heavy whipping cream (optional- if used add 4 GR);
- 1 tsp vanilla extract;
- 1 tsp maple flavoring.

Directions:

1. Heat griddle with oil or waffle iron.
2. Whisk together all ingredients in a medium bowl adding the water small amounts at a time until you get the consistency needed.

3. Spoon onto griddle or waffle iron.

4. Cook until crisp.

5. Serve with butter, cinnamon and/or low-carb syrup but remember to add any additional carbs from the syrup.

36. CRUSTLESS QUICHE LORRAINE

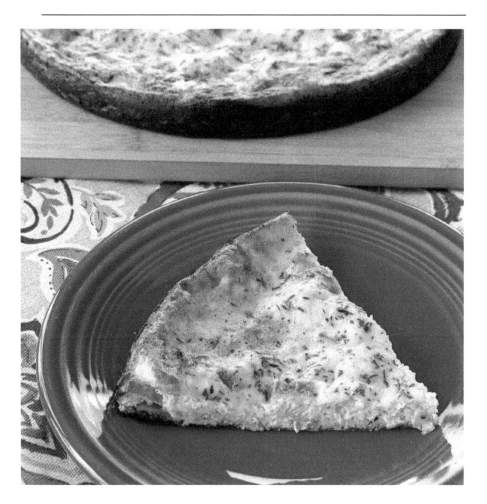

Ingredients:

- 5 eggs -- beaten
- 1 1/2 cups half & half or heavy cream
- 5 green onion -- snipped with scissors or small chopped onion

- ¼ green pepper chopped
- 1/2 cup spinach frozen or fresh
- 1/4 teaspoon salt
- 1/8 teaspoon pepper
- 3/4 cup bacon fried & crumbled
- 1 1/2 cups cheese (Cheddar, or Monterey, Swiss)

Directions:

Preheat oven to 350*

1. In lg. bowl beat eggs, add cream, mix.
2. Add all other ingredients and mix well. Pour egg mixture into a greased 9" or 10 " pie plate.
3. Place pie plate into a large baking dish and pour HOT water into the dish around the pie plate to a depth of 1 inch.
4. Bake quiche in the oven for 50 min. or until a knife inserted near center comes out clean.
5. Remove from oven.
6. Let stand for ten min.

37. CONFETTI SCRAMBLED EGGS

Ingredients:

- 3 eggs
- 1 Tbsp butter or olive oil
- 2 Tbsp chopped onion
- 2 Tbsp green bell pepper
- 1 Tbsp red bell pepper
- 2 ounce cheddar cheese
- 2 Tbsp chopped tomato (or salsa)
- 1 Tablespoon bacon bits

Directions:

1. In a small pan, melt butter (or add olive oil), add onion and bell pepper.
2. Cook till veggies are tender, add eggs.
3. Scramble till eggs are partially set, add the cheese.
4. Once done, remove from pan.
5. Sprinkle the tomato and bacon bits over the top.

38.   EGG-IN-A-POT

Ingredients:

- 1 whole egg
- heavy cream
- 0.5 oz ham, sliced in small strips
- 0.5 oz grated cheddar
- any (fresh) herbs to taste
- salt
- pepper1tsp olive oil

Directions:

1. Grease an ovenproof ramekin with the olive oil.
2. Carefully break the egg into the ramekin, taking care not to break the yoke.
3. Add the ham and cheese and any herbs if you want.
4. Top up with the heavy cream to about a third of an inch below the rim of the ramekin.
5. Bake in a preheated oven of 350 degrees for about 20-25 minutes.

39. SAUSAGE GRAVY

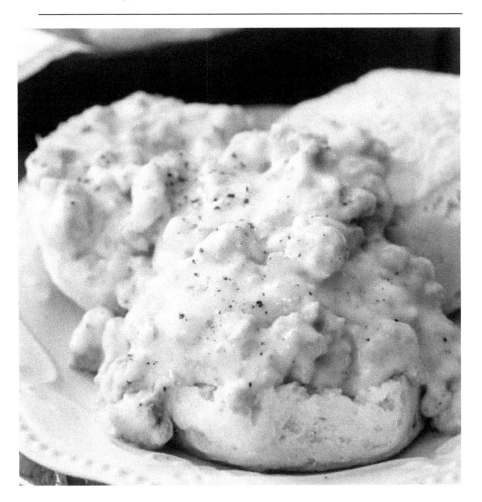

Ingredients:

- One roll of any breakfast sausage
- Approx 1/4 cup of water
- 1/2 teaspoon guar gum if necessary
- One pint of heavy whipping cream
- 1 egg

- salt and pepper to taste

Directions:

1. In a large skillet fry sausage until done.
2. Do not remove any of the grease from frying.
3. Turn down to low heat.
4. In a separate bowl whisk heavy cream and one egg together.
5. Add to the pan of sausage.
6. Salt and pepper to taste. You may need to add a small amount of water if it becomes too thick. Serve over low carb biscuits or eggs.
7. Entire recipe should be about 6-7 carbs or less and is wonderful.

40. BLT RANCH OMELET

Ingredients:

- 2 each large eggs
- 1 tablespoon water
- 2 tablespoons shredded cheddar cheese
- 3 slices bacon -- cooked crisp and crumbled
- 1/2 small tomato -- sliced thin
- 1/2 cup shredded lettuce
- 1 tablespoon mayonnaise
- 1 tablespoon salsa

Directions:

1. Beat eggs with a fork and add water, beat again to mix.
2. Add salt and pepper if desired and beat into egg.
3. Heat bacon drippings and pour egg mixture into small, non-stick pan.
4. Cook over low heat until set and no longer wet looking.
5. Pile bacon, cheese, lettuce and tomato on one half and flip the other half over to cover.
6. Remove from heat and cover pan for 30 seconds to melt cheese.
7. Mix salsa and mayo and spread over omelette.

41.   BREAKFAST BLT ROLL-UPS

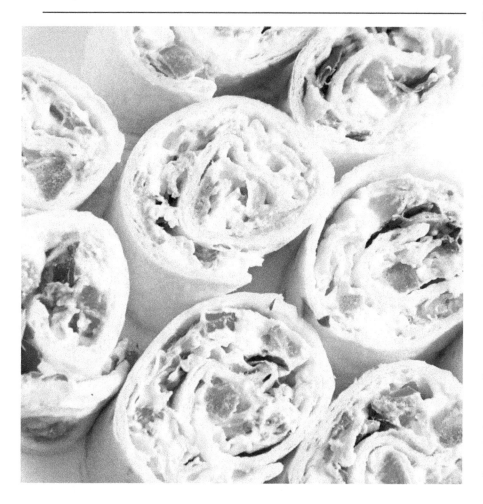

Ingredients:

- 4 each romaine lettuce leaves
- 1 tablespoon mayonnaise
- 3 slices bacon -- cooked crisp and crumbled
- 4 tablespoons shredded cheddar cheese
- 1/2 small roma tomato -- diced

Directions:

1. Shred 2 of the romaine leaves.
2. Mix shredded lettuce, mayo, cheese, bacon and tomato.
3. Add a little salt and pepper to taste.
4. Fill remaining 2 romaine leaves w/mixture, fold and enjoy.

42. WONDER WAFFLES

Ingredients:

- 2 Tbls. heavy cream
- 2 Tbls. water (0 carbs)
- 1 Tsp. vanilla extract
- 2 Pkt. Splenda (or 2 tsp. powdered Splenda)
- 2 or 3 ounces of crushed pork rinds
- 1/4 Tsp. ground cinnamon
- 3 Tbls. melted butter

Directions:

1. Beat the eggs then add the cream, water, and vanilla extract and beat some more.
2. Mix the Splenda with the cinnamon and then add that to the eggs.
3. When well blended mix in the ground pork rinds.
4. Let the mixture sit for a couple of minutes until it thickens. Then stir and check the consistency.
5. It should be quite thick, but not to thick to spoon easily. If too thick, add a little water.
6. If too thin, add a little bit more pork rinds.

7. Just before you're ready to put into waffle iron, stir in about 2/3 of the melted butter.

43. MOCK DANISH

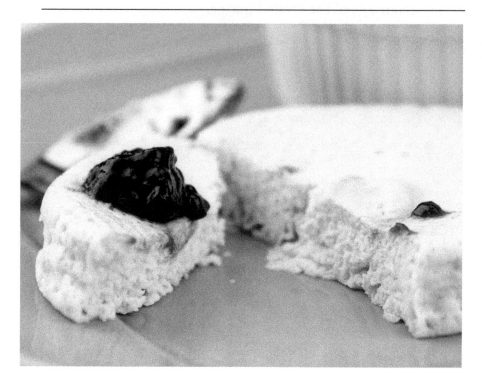

Ingredients:

- 3 oz cream cheese
- 1 egg, beaten
- 1/4 tsp vanilla extract
- dash of cinnamon
- 1 packet Splenda

Directions:

1. Heat the cream cheese in a small saucepan at low-medium heat till it is melted and creamy, stirring constantly.

2. Then, add the beaten egg, and begin whisking the mixture to really mix it well.
3. It will thicken as it cooks.
4. Continue whisking it, to keep it smooth.
5. When it starts to thicken, add the sweetener and seasonings.
6. Let it cook until it is very thick, thicker than pudding.
7. When it holds its shape on a spoon, it's done.
8. Chill and eat.

44. MEDITERRANEAN FRITTATA

Ingredients:

- 8 pitted kalamata olives (black olives will do in a pinch)
- 1 med. zucchini, cut into 1/2" cubes (about 2 cups)
- 1 sweet red pepper, diced
- 1/2 cup chopped onion
- 1/4 cup olive oil9 large eggs, lightly beaten
- 1/2 (4 ounce) package crumbled feta cheese
- 1/3 cup thinly sliced fresh basil
- 1/2 tsp salt
- 1/2 tsp freshly ground pepper
- 1/3 cup freshly grated Parmesan cheese
- basil sprigs for garnish

Directions:

1. Cook first 4 ingredients in hot oil in a 10" ovenproof skillet over med-high heat, stirring constantly, until vegetables are tender.
2. Combine eggs and next 4 ingredients; pour into skillet over vegetables.
3. Cover and cook over med-low heat 10 to 12 minutes or until almost set.
4. Remove from heat, and sprinkle with Parmesan cheese.

5. Broil 5 1/2" from heat (with electric oven door partially opened) 2 to 3 minutes or until golden.
6. Cut frittata into wedges; garnish, if desired.
7. Serve warm or at room temperature.

45. BREAKFAST EGG CASSEROLE

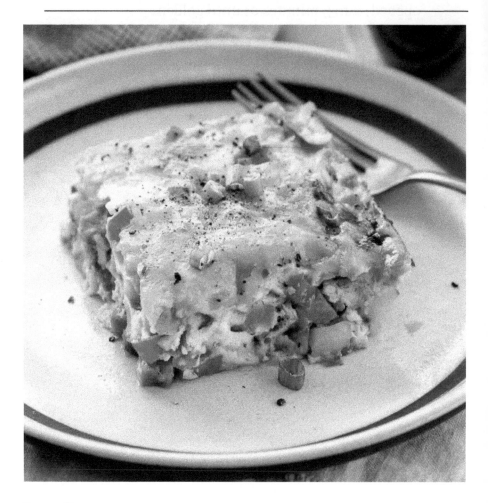

Ingredients:

- 6-12 eggs
- 1/2 cup crumpled bacon
- salt and pepper to taste
- garlic powder to taste1/4 cup onion
- 1/4 cup hot peppers (option)

- 1/2 cup broccoli (option)
- 2 tbsp heavy cream

Directions:

1. In a 9x13 pan mix all with a whisk.
2. Bake at 350 for 20-30 mins depending on how many eggs.
3. When done set slices of cheese to melt.
4. When cool, slice into 9 slice and freeze the rest for another day

46.   SWEET INDUCTION
BREAKFAST

Ingredients:

- 1/2 tablespoon butter
- 2 eggs
- 2 packets artificial sweetener2 tablespoons cream cheese
- 1 teaspoon heavy cream
- 1/2 teaspoon vanilla

Directions:

1. Heat frying pan and allow butter to coat the bottom.
2. Mix the 2 eggs with a packet of sweetener in a small bowl and pour into frying pan.
3. In another small bowl mix the cream cheese, heavy cream, vanilla and a packet of sweetener.
4. When the eggs are cooked, you can let them cool before adding the cream mixture or let the mixture melt slightly onto the warm eggs.
5. Gently spread the cream mixture to cover the eggs (like tomato sauce on a pizza).
6. Using a spatula roll the egg "crepe" together like a jelly roll.

47.   PORRIDGE

Ingredients:

- 1 egg
- 2 teaspoons protein powder -- soy, unflavoured half and half
- 1/4 cup powdered nuts (macadamia -- walnut, whatever)
- Sweetener

Directions:

1. As a note, just put the nuts into a blender and let it run enough to chop them into a coarse powder.
2. Mix the protein powder and the egg in a small mixing bowl. Add an equivalent volume of half and half, or cream.
3. Mix. Put the bowl in the microwave and cook on high for 1 1/2 minutes.
4. Mix again, and cook for 1 minute.
5. Adjust the time so that the mixture is cooked and not runny.
6. Mix again until it has the consistency of porridge. Mix in the nuts.
7. Add sweetener to taste, and add half and half as typical on porridge.
8. The result is pretty adequate with a slight eggy taste.

48.   BANANA NUT PORRIDGE

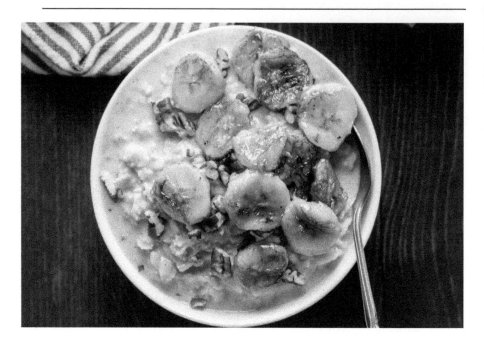

Ingredients:

- 2 Eggs
- 2 tablespoons water
- 2 tablespoons heavy cream
- 2 teaspoons sweetener
- 1 tablespoon psyllium
- husks1 tablespoon butter
- 1/2 cap vanilla flavoring
- 1/2 cap banana flavoring
- 1 good shake cinnamon
- 1 light shake nutmeg

Directions:

1. Beat all the ingredients, leaving 1 tbl cream and 1 tsp sweetener as topping.
2. Melt the butter in a skillet over medium heat, pour in the egg mixture.
3. Fold about 3 or 4 times. When the eggs just set, remove from heat & then put into bowl.
4. Sprinkle the remaining sweetener & add cream over the top.
5. In OWL a tbl of chopped Walnuts is nice.

49. SWEET CINNAMON PANCAKE

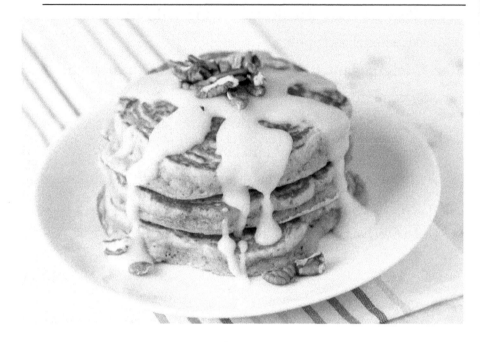

Ingredients:

- 2 eggs
- 1 ounce cream cheese
- 2 splenda packets -- (2 to 3)1 teaspoon heavy cream
- 1 teaspoon cinnamon -- (1 to 2)
- butter

Directions:

1. Melt cream cheese in microwave.
2. Mix in eggs, splenda, cream and cinnamon.
3. Melt butter on a frying pan and pour mixture

50.   FRENCH TOAST RECIPE

Ingredients:

- Two whole eggs
- tsp cinnamon
- 1 tbsp of Splenda granular or 1 packet of Splenda

Directions:

1. Combine ingredients.
2. Preheat skillet over medium heat and add 2 tbsp of Life Services High Oleic Sunflower Oil.
3. Beat mixture thoroughly with a fork and dip sliced Keto Cinnamon Bread in batter and fry until golden brown.
4. Enjoy with Keto Syrup and/or Betta Butta.

51. BREAKFAST BREAD

Ingredients:

- 1/4 cup protein powder
- 1/2 cup carbo-lite bake mix
- 1/4 cup flax seeds – ground into 1/2C meal
- 3 large eggs
- 1/2 cup sour cream1/4 cup water
- 1/2 teaspoon salt
- 2 teaspoons baking powder
- 3 tablespoons melted
- butter

Directions:

1. Preheat oven to 350f. Spray a standard 8" loaf pan (or an 8x8x2 cake pan) with cooking spray.
2. Mix dry ingredients in a large bowl.
3. Beat eggs with a fork and blend in butter, water and sour cream. Stir into dry ingredients until just blended.
4. Pour into prepared pan and bake: 30 minutes for square pan and 40 minutes for loaf pan.
5. This bread is semi-sweet because the carbo-lite bake mix has splenda in it.

52. TURKEY CLUB OMELETTE

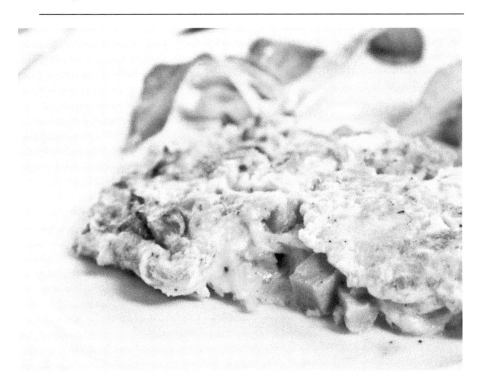

Ingredients:

- 3 Eggs
- 1/4 cup cubed turkey breast meat
- 2 strips bacon – cooked and chopped
- 2 tablespoons sour cream2 sprigs chives – coarsely chopped
- 2 slices tomato slices -- chopped
- 1/4 cup hollandaise sauce

Directions:

1. Prep all of your ingredients ahead of time.
2. Cook the eggs on one side and flip to other side.
3. Add ingredients and fold or roll.
4. Add hollandaise sauce over the top of omelette.

53. WAGON WHEEL FRITTATA

Ingredients:

- 1 tablespoon cooking oil
- 10 ounces frozen broccoli spears
- 1 tablespoon water
- 4 ounces button mushrooms -- drained
- 6 eggs2 tablespoons heavy cream
- 3 tablespoons water
- 1 1/2 teaspoons Italian seasoning -- crushed
- 6 thin tomato slices -- about
- 1 med tomato
- 1/4 cup grated Parmesan cheese

Directions:

1. In a 10-inch omelet pan or skillet over medium heat, combine oil, broccoli, and water.
2. Cover and cook just until broccoli can be broken apart with a fork, about 3 minutes.
3. Take pan off the heat.
4. Arrange broccoli spears so stems point to center of pan.
5. Set mushrooms, rounded sides up, between broccoli spears.

6. In medium bowl, thoroughly blend eggs, milk, and seasoning.
7. Pour over broccoli.
8. Cover and cook over medium heat until eggs are almost set.
9. Remove from heat.

54. TURKEY AND HAM FRITTATA

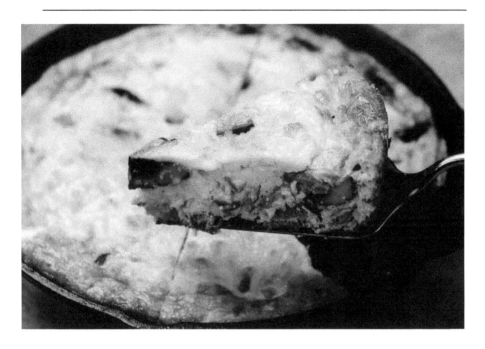

Ingredients:

- 1 cup chopped cooked turkey
- 1 cup chopped ham
- 6 eggs
- 3 tablespoons oil
- 2 medium tomatoes --
- chopped1 cup button mushroom -- diced
- 4 shallots -- chopped
- 1/2 cup heavy cream
- salt and ground black pepper for seasoning

Directions:

1. Put oil in large frying pan, add turkey, ham and mushrooms until mushrooms are tender.
2. Add tomatoes and onions.
3. Cook, stirring for 2 minutes.
4. In a bowl whisk together eggs, cream and seasoning, then pour into turkey and ham mixture in pan.
5. Cook gently until mixture is firm - the top will not be quite set.
6. Place pan under a hot griller to complete cooking the top for approx. 2 minutes.
7. Turn frittata on board and cut into wedges.
8. This recipe is great when you have all that leftover turkey and ham.

Lightning Source UK Ltd.
Milton Keynes UK
UKHW020638140621
385477UK00005B/31